14-9

Grady
Stay Safe
Jimi

1

NOTICE

DISCLAIMER

The information presented within this book represents solely view of the author and publishers and is intended for informational purposes only as of the date of publication. The author is active in a number of healthcare domains, and this book does not represent the view of the author's organizational associations. The use of "we" is a substitute for "I" in all cases.

This book offers no private or professional advice. The reader is encouraged to use good judgment when applying the information herein contained and to seek advice from a qualified professional, if needed. The author the and publishers shall in no event be held liable for any loss or other damages, including but not limited to special, incidental, consequential, or other damages. The reader is responsible for any subjective decision made as to the content and/or its use.

For questions or comments regarding any aspects of this book, Dr. Blair welcomes you to contact him at drjdblair@comcast.net.

4

TABLE OF CONTENTS

Author's Notes to a Trusting Public

Myths and realities face us each day. Diversify your 401K and you're sure to have a nest egg when you need it. Get that college education and you'll have job security. Work hard and gain experience, and you will reap your just rewards in your golden years.

Disappointments associated with evolving realities of these myths are full of angst, frustration and sorrow. However, they pale by comparison when measured against the myths and realities discussed in this book.

The author came out of semi-retirement on September 12, 2001. Soon after the shock of those devastating terrorist attacks had been internalized, it was replaced with a passion to contribute to the national effort to prepare for and respond to likely future attacks.

Past remembrances of combat mass

casualty scenes, ankle-deep in blood and facing the reality that all could not be saved, was an excruciatingly painful experience on a distant battlefield. The reality that it could happen at home is stuff for sleepless nights.

Up close and personal experiences dealing with Euro-terrorism (Red Brigade-Badder – Mienhoff) attacks on military and civilian populations demonstrated the vulnerability of soft targets, even in an environment in which the "culture of preparedness" is a way of life.

A decade of "boots on the ground" working with healthcare organizations across the nation to prepare for any number of natural and man-made threats has been professionally challenging. Along with the satisfaction such activities bring, one is also exposed to the extent that preparedness gaps exist in the greater healthcare system.

I liken it to a real-life "myth buster

exercise." To my admiration for Alexander Pope's "To err is human; to forgive, divine," I would add; "Trust not yourself, but your defects to know, make use of every friend and foe."

This book is written for the trusting public. Reasonable expectations for meaningful change must include the consumer's spirited advocacy for any healthcare product, including a safe and secure locus of care.

Repeated exposures to Agent Orange and other "slings and arrows of outrageous (mis) fortune" have taken their toll. Life-limiting conditions have added to the author's sense of urgency to close the gaps; yet, working together, we can make it happen.

The last page of this book, "Why This is So Important," tells it all.

JB

"In the coming months, another terror attempt on U.S. soil is certain."

U.S. Intelligence Chiefs, February 3, 2010

"New Terrorism Risk Review Released Friday"

"Lack of Hospital Surge Capacity Still a Problem"

"Rules on World's Most Deadly Pathogens Could Be Revised"

"FBI Director: Somali Jihadists Could Launch Attacks in U.S."

"Inept Nurses Free to Work in New Locales"

"Earthquake Fault Much Larger, More Dangerous Than Thought"

"Pakistan Taliban Leader Threatens Attacks On U.S. Cities"

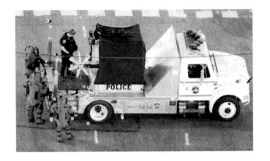

Close Call – April 2010

INTRODUCTION

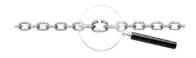

Early searching for this book title was a struggle in itself. More than five decades in healthcare have taught the author that things are not always as they appear. Where one stands on evolving issues is largely a function of where you sit. Past vivid memories are colored by perceptions of success and disappointments along the way.

Traveling through a professional lifetime in which the nation has faced threats from nation states first, and later from non-state actors bearing the same set of weapons, Weapons of

Mass Destruction (WMD), has provided an ever-present background with a need to be prepared to respond when dangers come. Cultural changes across those years are indeed significant, none more significant than the locus and manner in which hospital and healthcare is offered.

The healthcare delivery system has morphed from its altruistic, patient-centered roots into a highly competitive, bottom-line, impersonal commercial business. This does not mean that today's hospital systems do not have altruistic, dedicated folks. However, they have limited influence on current delivery of care.

Ten years ago, the Institute of Medicine's (IOM) startling report, "To Err is Human," served as a catalyst to address mounting life-threatening dangers in the nation's hospitals. The report revealed alarming, widespread patient safety issues, including hospital acquired infections (HAI) and a shocking number of patient care errors euphemistically called "medical misadventures."

The May 2009 Consumer Reports publication took a look at the intervening decade in the nation's crusade against the curse of healthcare treatment-related misadventures. It is their opinion that the ten-year initiative had done little to change the approximately 100,000 avoidable deaths in the nation's healthcare system and the millions of treatment errors which inflict injury and suffering on those passing through that system.

The intense focus on this dimension of patient safety and security has significantly increased the use of human and financial resources. Over the years, this patient safety and security function has essentially morphed into an almost exclusive clinical domain.

The noble goals of access, quality and affordability have been healthcare challenges for decades. The 21st century is filled with the possibility of unimagined advances in our ability to achieve those noble goals and make our citizens healthier and longer-lived.

Shadowing that optimistic future are more frequent and robust natural disasters, evolving infectious diseases and other dark, sinister forces poised to destroy that future, and at its most terrifying a combination of these forces. This book addresses the other side of patient safety and security and the consequences of healthcare industry's lack of attention to homeland security healthcare readiness. Purported to be one of the most regulated industries in the country, it also holds the rarely disputed title of "weakest link in the homeland security chain."

Who, then, is watching the vulnerable hospital and healthcare emergency management store?

Not unlike the Institute of Medicine's "To Err is Human," a rude national wake-up call for quality and safety in the nation's hospitals and healthcare delivery communities, other national wake-up calls, the 9/11 attacks, and the Gulf Coast killer hurricane Katrina have resulted in poor responses and the same message: "To err is human – to delay is deadly."

If past is prologue, it teaches us that Americans are reluctant to prepare for known or perceived existential threat. This propensity for reactive rather than proactive behavior is legion and alive and well in today's healthcare delivery system.

The familiar mantra to the improvement of healthcare for the masses, "an ounce of prevention is worth a pound of cure," fills the halls of Congress during the current debates on how to reform our healthcare system. However, at the end of the day, profitable intervention always trumps the more valuable course of prevention.

The post cold war strategy for homeland security protection has its roots in the concern that the feared weapons of mass destruction (WMDs) may well fall into the hands of known, and yet unknown, non-state terrorists.

Many date the modern post cold war WMD threat with President Reagan's November 1988 Executive Order 12656: Assignment of Emergency Preparedness Responsibilities. The Department of Health and Human Services (DHHS) was tasked with the development of a comprehensive national healthcare plan to mobilize the nation's healthcare industry to meet the immediate challenges posed by these emerging terrorist threats.

The principles that guide the national strategy for homeland security are found in a plethora of statutes, executive orders, and presidential directives, homeland security presidential directives spanning decades. Today, the roadmap for a comprehensive strategy for homeland security is found in the National Response Framework (NRF) along with its companion document, the National Incident Management System (NIMS). Together, they serve as a guide to how the nation conducts a unified all-hazards response.

The over-arching theme imbedded in the NRF and NIMS is a concept of good-faith partnership between and among the nation's economic sectors; federal, public, private, tribal, and non-governmental. The planning goal is to build a seamless bulwark against natural and man-made threats (all-hazards).

Despite these directives, the nation's healthcare sector finds itself ill-prepared to deal with known threats to the safety and security of the country. This lack of comprehensive preparedness places us all at risk. Perhaps the greatest disparity is found in the difference between the actual level of hospital and healthcare preparedness and a trusting public's perception of that preparedness.

In the following chapters, we will explore existing serious healthcare gaps by looking at urban, suburban, exurban and rural myths, and the soft underpinning of those misguided perceptions.

"The history of man is a graveyard of great cultures that came to catastrophic ends because of their incapacity for planning rational, voluntary reaction to challenge."

Eric Fromm

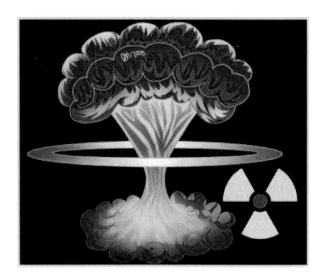

CHAPTER 1: MYTH 1

The Nation's Healthcare Community is Prepared to Respond to an Increasingly Hostile Environment.

Reality: The non-federal healthcare sector with its public/private blend faces the usual set of regulatory requirements. Effective oversight of the healthcare industry has always been challenging. In a free pluralistic healthcare industry, governance is a fragmented and a very complex undertaking. Preparing the nation's healthcare delivery system to cope with nature's threats is formidable. Adding the possible permutations of creative terrorist threats and newly emerging infectious diseases is mind-numbing.

State and tribal sovereignty and the stark dichotomy between federal health sectors mandatory and the non-federal health sectors voluntary compliance embedded in the National Response Framework (NRF) creates huge barriers to the realization of an effective national all-hazards response.

The federal healthcare delivery sector owns and operates approximately ten percent (10%) of the nation's healthcare delivery capacity. The bulk, upward to ninety percent (90%), of the nation's healthcare delivery resources is owned and operated by the non-federal sector. This sector has shown little appetite to meet its expected roles and responsibilities on a voluntary basis. Influential segments of the health sector have done little to advocate for or to facilitate a realistic movement toward an effective level of participation.

This attitude of denial, apathy, and cognitive dissonance within the operating segment of the industry is a continuing disappointment. It takes more than an inattentive hospital industry and its immediate support system to leave an entire economic sector ill-prepared to meet known challenges.

Lack of strong Department of Homeland Security (DHS) leadership and a poorly coordinated Department of Health and Human Services (DHHS) cross-agency, hand-off of major responsibilities resulted in a lackluster start. Leadership at state administrative levels, combined with state legislative bodies unwilling to provide enabling legislative actions to remove legal, ethical and moral barriers has retarded the development of a cohesive national healthcare response. Add a seemingly indifferent, non-federal healthcare industry into this mix, and one gets a healthcare sector seriously behind the power curve.

The enormous size and disparate functions represented in this industry, which employees over 13 million individuals, helps one to understand the challenges inherent in assembling them into an effective partnership for homeland security protection. Over a half-million establishments make up the industry. Hospitals and medical centers represent only 2% of the facilities; however, they employ 40% of the human resources.

About 76% of healthcare facilities are offices of physicians, dentists, or other health practitioners. The private healthcare sectors are found in the following broad functional areas:

- Approximately 6,000 hospitals of varying sizes
- More than 492,000 ambulatory health facilities
- Nearly 70,000 nursing and residential care facilities
- Nearly 175,000 individual or group medical practices
- Over 100 health insurance companies

- More than 40,000 pharmacies
- Approximately 2,500 pharmaceutical manufacturers, some international
- Large medical devices and supplies industries
- More than 500 blood and organ bank establishments
- More than 30,000 funeral directors

The development of a viable healthcare sector prepared to respond to all-hazards depends on leadership planning and cooperation at all levels of oversight.

"Study: Terrorists Shifting Focus to Soft Targets"

"MI5 Discover Al Qaeda Buying Ambulances on eBay"

"Obama Likely to Go Slow on Homeland Security Issues"

"Prepare for an Attack"

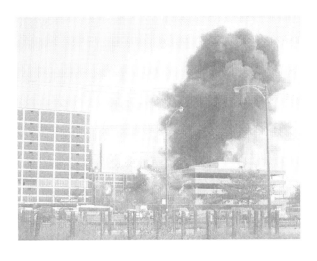

CHAPTER 2: MYTH 2

Hospitals and Healthcare Facilities are Unlikely Targets
for Terrorist Attacks.

Reality: This society acts as if hospitals are immune to terrorist attacks. Hospitals may well be seen as soft and desirable targets by those who may wish to do us harm. The killing and injuring of mass numbers of patients, caregivers, and others in an urban-clustered medical center and the contemporaneous loss of that resource to respond would undoubtedly create a terror multiplier effect (TME). The cascading effects of such an event would push mass casualty care to surrounding healthcare facilities less well-prepared for the task.

Unlike geographic bound disasters, such as hurricanes and earthquakes, these events terrorize the national population; much like an approaching hurricane in the Gulf Coast terrifies those in its path. However, the same level of fear and anxiety probably will not be felt by the corn farmer in Nebraska.

Following on the heels of the 9/11 terrorist attacks, the nation's urban medical centers were alerted by the Federal Bureau of Investigation (FBI) that the next set of terrorist attacks would be aimed at their facilities. The Veterans Administration was also notified that their hospitals were viewed by terrorists as soft and vulnerable military targets. The prevailing thought that at-risk targets were seen as closely associated with known geographic areas may or may not be an appropriate determinant for sector critical infrastructure protection.

A series of unexplained intrusions into hospitals across the nation is the cause of significant concern among all terrorism experts. Most often occurring in the middle of the night, visits by individuals with fraudulent credentials seeking facility tours and detailed information on locations of pharmaceutical stockpiles, nuclear medical clinics, and other sensitive operational infrastructure is unsettling. The size, geography, and ownership of these facilities did not demonstrate any common pattern, other than that they were hospitals.

Less intrusive events dealt with theft of hospital paraphernalia, laboratory coats, and identification tags. Purchase of used ambulances and theft of emergency vehicles appeared to be replaced by reproduction. The use of these vehicles as delivery platforms for future terrorist attacks is of considerable concern. The non-federal clustered urban medical centers are particularly vulnerable to this attack mode.

Worldwide examples of the vulnerability of hospitals to any manner of terrorist attacks are documented in a plethora of anti/counter terrorism archives, some open-sourced, others classified. Some have been simply brazen attacks by terrorists walking into the hospital and killing patients.

Truck and car bombs have been very effective. Some terrorists have resorted to suicide bombers masquerading as patients, while others have been targets of opportunity killed in the ambulance-to-entrance space. Recent attacks on hospitals in India have almost escaped our national attention. One-fifth of the Mumbai terrorist force attacked the city's Cama Hospital, the third such attacks on hospitals in the region.

It may be well for us to reflect on terrorists attacks in Russia. The last decade of the 20th Century was a violent period for Russia in their struggle with Chechen terrorism. They had been able to deal with deadly attacks in multiple sites within the country, massive urban attacks, buried Cesium 137 devices, school attacks, rail bombing, and other attacks. Only one attack changed the nature of the conflict and was seen as a major success for the terrorists; the event, the Budyonnovsk hospital hostage crisis with its 200 deaths.

"We shape our buildings; thereafter, they shape us."

Winston Churchill

"Five Lessons U.S. Hospitals Can Take from Haiti"

"Construction: Eight Complexes are Unsafe, According to the State"

"California Hospitals Seek Relief from Seismic Safety Rules"

"San Francisco Identifies Building Most At Risk"

"Baja Quake Impact Reaches California"

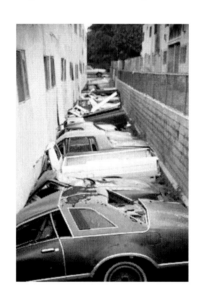

CHAPTER 3: MYTH 3

The Non-Federal Healthcare Sector has Followed the Federal Healthcare Sector in All-Hazards Design and Construction of its Facilities.

Reality: As federal and metropolitan governments build more robust structures and mitigate safety and security vulnerabilities in their building environments, non-federal structures become more susceptible to terrorist attacks. Experts tell us that approximately 25% of all target selection is opportunity.

Along with the national strategy for physical protection of Critical Infrastructure and Key Assets (CI/KA) and earlier actions to fortify federal structures against anticipated terrorist attacks, Presidential Decision Directive (PPD 63) gained a high profile after the bombing of the Oklahoma City federal Murrah Building. The major focus of these initiatives is to prepare for possible terrorist attacks using weapons of mass destruction (WMD). The Oklahoma City domestic attack infused a sense of urgency into the effort. The current initiatives are found in the National Infrastructure Protection Plan (NIPP).

The federal healthcare sector has followed initiatives to protect against all known hazardous threats through designing, constructing, and retrofitting its healthcare facilities and the application of timely "lessons learned" action strategies. These actions have mitigated many of the existing vulnerabilities from a range of known natural and man-made threats. As a result, the workplace environment for the federal healthcare workforce is measurably safer and more secure than its non-federal counterpart.

A quick review of GAO-10-436, Defense

Infrastructure, will provide the reader with better understanding of challenges posed by current expectations of Design and Construction outcomes with the competing goals of cost containment, sustainability, and anti-terrorism protection.

The history of the non-federal healthcare sector meeting its expected homeland security roles and responsibilities through voluntary compliance has been dismal. The non-federal healthcare sector designs and constructs its hospital facilities without taking full advantage of known opportunities for the dual benefits of aggressive vulnerability reduction into its facilities.

The 2006 American Institute of Architects (AIA) Healthcare Design and Construction Guidance for Healthcare Facilities is the industry's professional "bible" for hospital and healthcare construction. It is basically silent on mitigation of vulnerabilities associated with today's known threats.

Guidance to the healthcare industry is updated and published every four years. The organization works with a variety of regulatory and advisory bodies to develop, review and promulgate standards, codes and guidelines.

The 2002 Edition was written as if the nation were still enjoying the halcyon days of the peace dividend. Five years after the 9/11 terrorist attacks and a year after the Katrina tragedy, the 2006 Edition evidenced little change in guidance. The first review of the document left many incredulous. We were disappointed in the lack of attention to the changing threat landscape.

A series of interviews with those who contributed to the document left us scratching our heads and looking for some answers. The official answer says it all: "... would like to state that all 125 committee members are dedicated to making the Guidelines for Design and Construction of Healthcare Facilities a top-notch set of recommended standards…." There is not a person on the committee that has intentionally tried to keep any effort to add language for "hardening our healthcare buildings out of the guidelines." At the time, we attempted, without success, to find evidence that the Department of Homeland Security had been involved in the review process.

The healthcare construction industry has enjoyed a recent building boom, which rivals the early Hill-Burton Hospital construction era. These healthcare work sites house healthcare stakeholders who will be providing care for the next two generations.

The opportunity that was lost to reduce vulnerability to both natural and man-made threats is incalculable. The healthcare industry must accept the notion that hospitals and other healthcare organizations are involved in almost every classification of all-hazards threats.

There is a case to be made for priority protection for healthcare facilities, in general, and hospitals in particular. All significant casualty-producing events involve timely actions by these organizations, either directly or indirectly.

To be as prepared as possible, it is a 24/7 responsibility to be prepared to care for all walking through their front doors, regardless of scale, origin, and nature of event. The hospital industry has turned a blind eye to one-half of its mission in a terrorist threat environment in the defense of its facilities and in the protection of its stakeholders. The most sophisticated mass casualty protocols and treatment modalities are only as good as the freedom to exercise them.

There is little need to discuss the role of design and construction in the sustainability of buildings in earthquake zones. The visual documentation of this year's earthquakes in Haiti, Chile and Turkey and their devastating aftermath leaves little chance to trump with the printed word.

These events clearly demonstrate the unbelievable chaos that accompanies earthquake disasters. They also illustrate the need for advanced preparedness and the indispensible need for a unified command structure. If everyone is in control, no one is in control.

Great numbers of folks ready to volunteer and huge piles of medical supplies and other items are necessary, but not sufficient, to respond to the immediate needs of suffering masses.

Earthquake zones in the U.S. have been identified. However, the U.S. Geological Survey folks, through no fault of their own, keep finding new earthquake fault connections. The

All-Hazards Preparedness and Response community is most concerned about earthquake zones located in densely populated areas like the American West Coast – California, Oregon, Washington, Alaska, Hawaii – and in the Middle West New Madrid Fault Line areas – Missouri, Tennessee, Illinois, Kentucky, Mississippi, Georgia, and South Carolina.

The coastal areas are also subject to the dual hazards of tsunamis. The destructive power of tsunamis has been visually documented through recent events in Indonesia, Malaysia, and Burma, with its death toll of over 230,000 individuals.

We cannot generalize hospital earthquake readiness based on concerns which have plagued this hospital industry in California. However, these concerns have surfaced repeatedly by those at risk in hospitals where structures have not been seismically upgraded.

Responding to the 1994 Northridge earthquake and the resulting damage to the area's hospitals, the State legislative body mandated a robust program to seismically upgrade the State's hospitals. It has been difficult to follow the political machinations by legislative actions. However, drop-dead dates for implementation of these seismic upgrades have had mixed results and leave many at risk.

A recent article in the Sacramento Bee leaves one with the impression that the "dust has not settled on the issue," as evidenced in the caption, "California hospitals seek relief from seismic safety rules." The California Hospital Association has petitioned to throw out the 2013 upgrade mandates.

The California Nurses Association (CNA) is and has been a strong voice for action. They indicate that one-half of the existing hospitals need to be seismically upgraded. Other studies indicate that 47% of hospital floor space needing upgrades are in the Los Angeles and San Francisco Bay areas. We see little value in sharing the projected numbers of deaths and serious injuries, should the earth adjust its plates in this region. As a non-lawyer, we will not speculate on the level of risk exposure this scenario represents.

Since disparate groups are at loggerheads about how society deals with the many arcane legal, ethical, and moral judgments in protection of a trusting public, it seems necessary that these disparities must be put aside in the face of these obvious dangers. Long-time observers say that the current argument that funds are not available in "lean times" rings hollow, seeing that they were not made available during earlier fat times.

The existence of what the nurses call an Occupational Safety and Health Act (OSHA) violation in "known unsafe workplaces" does not appear to impact on DHHS (conditions of participation) or "deemed status" eligibility to receive payment for the care of federal beneficiaries. The same may be said for selection as one of the "best of breed" from the growing cottage industry of a hundred best of "this and that." Organizations that presume to guide a trusting public to the best quality and safety for healthcare should take great care to factor in physical safety of that locus of care.

"Mumbai Attacks Refocus U.S. Cities"

"Overlooked: The Littlest Evacuees"

"Sleeper Hezbollah Cells Have Reawakened"

"Hospital Settles in Katrina-related Case"

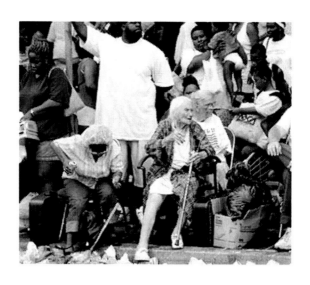

CHAPTER 4: MYTH 4

Federal Help is On The Way to Support the Unready.

Reality: The several states are responsible for the health, safety and security of their populations. For the most part, all-hazard events are local. Local and/or regional communities are expected to successfully prepare and respond to their emergencies, and hospital authorities are expected to prepare for and respond to disasters using their own and coordinated community resources.

The most immediate decision to be made by hospital authorities facing all-hazards events is fundamental to the survival, lives, and health of all stakeholders: protect in place or evacuate.

An informed decision to protect in place is just that, and timely information on patient census and the likely surge of patients and others seeking safe harbor are essential. The levels of essential medications in an era of "just in time deliveries" (food and other supplies for the current and expected population) must be made available for the anticipated length of a disaster event. Leaders must be kept informed of the expected impact on critical systems and readiness of back-up systems.

The decision for "evacuation" is no less complex. The availability of dependable transportation, safe and secure routes of evacuation, pre-designated alternative site capability of meeting the needs of evacuated patient populations and other stakeholders are but a few of the questions to be answered. Timely informed answers to these questions are not available in the middle of a disaster ("you can't change the tires on a moving vehicle"). It requires thoughtful preplanning. The survival of an organization is in the hands of local planners. Assistance from outside responders may or may not make the scene in time to save the unready.

Under the category of "things do not always seem as they appear," the tragic deaths in New Orleans hospitals during hurricane Katrina provide us with an example of failure at all levels of government to protect the most vulnerable among us; frail/elderly inpatients, most on life support systems.

From all objective signs, the trusting citizens of New Orleans could be secure in the knowledge that their healthcare community was prepared to deal with hurricanes, which are the recognized greatest hazard in the area. A year before the killer storm, the region completed a million-dollar hurricane exercise (PAM). The exercise findings were a near "clone" to what was to take place in the future in the form of the Katrina hurricane.

All the major hospitals in the city had comforting signs of readiness – certifications and accreditations; all affirmations of their preparedness to deal with the region's most dangerous and most exercised natural hazard.

Hurricane Katrina was tracked by authorities for days prior to landfall. The storm's speed, strength, and every movement were available to hospital authorities and other official decision makers, with an hour-to-hour warning of the destructive path and the time and place for landfall. Hospital organizations made the decision to "protect in place." Many question the wisdom of that choice. The rest is history.

Many have chronicled the horror experienced by patients and caregivers in those critical days after the storm struck. Like clockwork, each year around the anniversary of that tragic event, there is a flurry of articles about the disaster.

A book published in November 2009, Nursing in Hell: The Katrina Experience, chronicles the day-by-day horrors experienced by nine nurses trapped in hospitals the week after Katrina. The author, nurse Marti Jordan, Ph.D., reports that she went through a lot of "soul searching" before she dared to proceed with her investigation, which would put the volunteer participants through what must have been times filled with fear and anguish. These brave caregivers and Dr. Jordan shared a vision that "lessons learned" from the interviews could one day spare others from their avoidable fate.

Some participants found the retelling of this experience therapeutic. Others found little relief in reliving those unspeakable days of agony and despair. Dr. Jordan has taken the book on the road with the hope that it will influence future decisions made by hospital authorities in critical life and death decisions. Her lecture series is entitled, "So It Will Never Happen Again."

The human cost to caregivers caught in these tragic circumstances may never be known. All participants in the study suffered from various degrees of post-traumatic stress disorder (PTSD).

The psychological cost to these brave caregivers is difficult to measure. The same may be said about the pain and suffering of patient victims and their loved ones. The cost to hospital and healthcare systems will be tallied after years of legal battles.

The most recent Katrina related death trial was settled three weeks into the proceedings. The case took a high profile in 2007, when the Louisiana Supreme Court decided that the family could seek damages under general liability, as opposed to malpractice claims, which is capped at one-half million dollars ($500,000.) The plaintiffs later sued the hospital owners for $11.7 million in the Orleans Parish Civil District Court, charging wrongful death.

The court sealed the trial records after the January 2010 settlement.

The impact of the settlement regarding legal exposure for hospitals as to their responsibility to prepare for and respond to known outside and inside threats is being followed closely by the industry. Consequently, the importance of hospital and healthcare organizations' preplanning and their ability to make informed decisions to "protect in place or evacuate" cannot be overstated.

Had terrorists taken advantage of the storm to seed any number of biological agents into the flooded areas, the casualty count would have been catastrophic. The terrorist community has observed the vulnerability created during all-hazards events and has identified tactics which may be used to coincide with these events.

Post Katrina investigators have surfaced concerns over questionable actions taken to safeguard critical chemical, biological and radiological materials, and additional accounting for infected research animals and other harmful toxins in the custody of hospitals, healthcare facilities, and research laboratories.

"W. PA. Bioterrorism Lab Fails Inspection"

"Bioterrorism's Threat Persists as Top Security Risk"

"Children Are Not Small Adults"

"H1N1: Pandemic or Not Pandemic?"

"Workers Imperiled by Lack of Pandemic Flu Readiness"

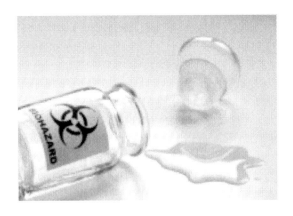

CHAPTER 5: MYTH 5

U.S. Hospitals are Prepared for Bioterrorism.

Reality: Three years and billions spent on federal initiatives to prepare for pandemic flu had a limited impact on the nation's readiness to deal with H1N1 (novel flu) pandemic. The disease had spread from Central Mexico to the United States before it was identified and effective cross-border defensive and protective measures came into play. Lack of robust border security and a weak surveillance tracking system made for a chaotic response.

Results from two hospital surveys which coincided with the time of the first wave notification of the novel flu found that almost

200 surveyed hospitals did not have written pandemic flu response plans. Reports of limited availability of personal protective equipment, protective masks, and other required supplies filled daily media accounts.

Availability of medical countermeasures, medications, and severe shortage of mechanical ventilators to treat advanced cases of the disease created a need for public guidance in the use of scarce medical supplies and equipment. Early H1N1 cases among caregivers threatened the surge capabilities of healthcare organizations.

Morbidity and mortality reports identified age-related cohorts at increased risk. Certain prison populations are among these groups. Commonly accepted methods for prevention and control of endemic and pandemic diseases are difficult to implement within incarceration environments. As a result, social distancing, limited isolation capacity, restrictions on items which may be introduced into the system, and a poor compliance place the group at high risk.

High background levels of chronic conditions, like HIV, TB and others, will increase the need for advanced treatment in these locations. Local hospitals that have prison contract agreements, emergency care beyond the capability of prison healthcare facilities, and all-hazards arrangements to support these populations during health related disasters are realistic planning concerns for all healthcare organizations.

Another identified group at high risk, infants and children, poses its own set of challenges. Infants and children are much more vulnerable to all these threats in our increasingly hostile world. Low dose exposures of chemical, biological, radiological and nuclear sources, which may cause minor disruptions among adults, may well be fatal among children.

Generally, acute care hospitals do not serve large pediatric populations and have limited capacity for expansion of care to this group. Community based facilities have limited supplies of critical resources, such as pharmaceuticals in pediatric doses and appropriately sized equipment, such as mechanical ventilators and other respiratory equipment (Ambu Mask). Too often, planners forget that kids are not miniature adults.

Federal guidance for "priority care and later priority vaccine recipients" from limited supplies were of great concern for authorities and made for some strange decision making; a case in point, parents asking authorities why the local prison received their H1N1 vaccines before the local school system.

The H1N1 second wave caught the nation flatfooted, unprepared for that event. Many have been highly critical of today's response to a known biological threat and an obvious breakdown in our ability to cope with and account for infectious events as they transpire.

Serious problems with the reliability of available tests, false-positive findings are disruptive and lead to waste of limited resources, and false-negative findings place whole populations at risk. The consequence of failure to recognize and measure the extent of H1N1 pandemic does not bode well for the future and has eroded public confidence in the system.

Regarding H1N1 versus bioterrorism, the 2009 WMD Commission, Graham/Talent Report surfaces new concerns over an old threat, bioterrorism. It posits "that the national attention to preparedness for bioterrorism has lost its vigor."

We have expressed our concern with the national movement away from bioterrorism preparedness to the more politically acceptable pandemic flu. The opportunities lost to achieve the dual benefits of being prepared for bioterrorism and to create a solid defense against evolving infectious diseases are incalculable. The news release Chicago, March 13, 2003 by the American College of Healthcare Executives (ACHE) stating, "Hospital CEOs say bioterrorism plans are in place," may have been premature.

Biological hazards for hospitals come from a number of sources. We have discussed the self-inflicted category in our discussion of hospital acquired infections (HAI). Endemic and pandemic infections may penetrate hospitals' defenses from the local community. Unexpected biological agents introduced either intentionally or by accident (bioterror/bioerror) into the environment are fraught with unimagined consequences.

Some speculate that the greatest national biological danger comes from the unbridled proliferation of bio laboratories across the country. An estimated 15,000 individuals work directly with these deadly agents. Proper vetting of these employees is an administrative challenge, and there is a fear that the potential gaps in disciplined background checks could result in serious "insider threats."

Hospital authorities must recognize the threat posed by these activities in their vicinities and develop a means to identify and respond to agent specific events. One of the greatest bio threats is where bio-agents are introduced into the hospital environment (bioterror/bioerror). Terrorists may well take advantage of endemic and pandemic events to introduce a different agent into the mix.

"Nuclear Waste Piles Up at Hospitals"

"Plutonium Spill, Laser Accident Prompt Reviews"

"FBI, Nuclear Agency Investigate Terrorism Suspect"

"The Little Nukes That Got Away"

"Dirty Bomb Recovery Plans Lacking"

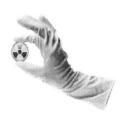 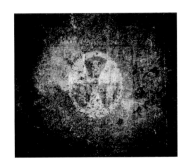

CHAPTER 6: MYTH 6

U.S. Hospitals are Ready to Deal with Nuclear and Radiological Threat.

Reality: Our first encounter with the "cesium 137 threat" to hospitals was during the background investigation of the terrorist physicians in the United Kingdom. The MI5, the U.K.'s intelligence organization, had gathered intelligence that non-state terrorists had identified "medical radioactive devices which could be used in the construction of a dirty bomb." The U.K. National Health Service took immediate action to harden these sites, restricting access by creating multiple layers of security, and in some cases removal of the cesium all together.

The U.S. Defense Science Board in their 2007 summer studies report labeled the cesium 137 containers found in approximately 1,000 medical facilities "low-hanging fruit," as half of the dreaded Radiological Disbursal Device (RDD) "dirty bomb."

An article, "Feds work to secure potential 'dirty bomb' source," surfaced in an August 2009 USA Today publication. Surprisingly, the issue was discussed in an open and cavalier manner with the astonishing revelation that, "The cesium 137 irradiator in one container would be enough for terrorists to make a radioactive bomb."

Accompanying this statement were the words, "red teams (friendly forces challenging security defenses of friendly sites) were able to defeat existing hospital defenses within two minutes, although there is no immediate or credible threat," a congressional homeland security subcommittee in a field briefing earlier this year was told that 40 of 840 cesium 137 containers had been hardened and "the rest will be hardened" between this 2010 and 2016.

In case this is one of those "to err is human" situations, it is useful to know that the cesium 137 contained in one container could be exploded in place, or stolen and exploded at a time and place of a terrorist's choice. The explosion and radioactive contamination could shut down 25 square kilometers at the site for 40 or more years, and clean-up costs would approach $1B per event.

Experts tell us that there should be a layered system of protection to secure these devices. The issue of "Is there a reasonable substitute for cesium 137?" has been raging in the scientific community for years. The thing we do know is that these devices present clear and present danger, and the healthcare community cannot have it both ways. If the healthcare community wants to keep them in the inventory, then they must secure them. Oversight of procurement and the use and security of medical use radioactive materials are of continuing concern for local communities.

According to the Nuclear Regulatory Commission report released in February 2008, 4,363 medical use radioactivity sources have been lost, stolen, or abandoned in the last decade.

Terrorism experts indicate that the issues over dirty bombs wax and wane over time. Recent attention has been given to rumors that Al Qaeda dirty bomb experts have returned to the United States.

GAO-06-826 – Disaster Preparedness: Limitations in Federal Evacuation Assistance for Health Facilities Should be Addressed

GAO-04-850 – Medicare: CMS Needs Additional Authority to Adequately Oversee Patient Safety in Hospitals

GAO-07-39 – Critical Infrastructure Protection: Progress Coordinating Government and Private Sector Efforts Varies by Sectors' Characteristics

GAO-08-539 – Influenza Pandemic: Federal Agencies Should Continue to Assist States to Address Gaps in Pandemic Planning

GAO-10-381T – Emergency Preparedness: State Efforts to Plan for Medical Surge Could Benefit from Shared Guidance for Allocating Scarce Medical Resources

GAO-10-436 – Defense Infrastructure: DOD Needs to Determine and Use the Most Economical Building Materials and Methods When Acquiring New Permanent Facilities

CRS-R40159 – Public Health and Medical Preparedness and Response: Issues in the 111th Congress

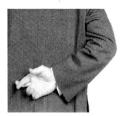 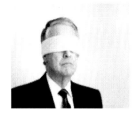

CHAPTER 7: MYTH 7

Public Health and Healthcare Sectors
"A Dynamic Duo"

Reality: Inside the All-Hazards Homeland Security Readiness Arena, the Public Health and Healthcare sector lags behind most of its economic sector counterparts. The coupling of public health and private public healthcare providers has had its legal, ethical, moral, communication, and philosophical problems. In many respects, they are the "odd couple."

The Public Health Service with its deep orientation to preventive medicine and bureaucratic stovepipe funding (underfunding) is an unlikely partner for the bottom-line oriented hospital, non-federal provider sector. The assumption is that the public health sector and the established, high profile, traditional "first responder community" would take the lead and coordinate committee planning with the non-federal healthcare provider groups.

The hospital-based healthcare provider responder groups were slow to be recognized as first responders and first receivers. As a consequence, the first responders funding was disproportionately distributed to public health and other seasoned first responder groups with traditional ties to existing federal and state "stovepipe funding mechanism." The non-federal healthcare national and state level trade organizations were reluctant supporters of the nation's strategy for homeland security, as were other segments of the industry.

The initial frenzy to do their part in the larger effort slowly cooled, as it became obvious that federal funds were limited. The old mantra of "unfunded mandates" filled the halls of Congress. Some preparedness funds trickled down from states, and some states felt that they were in a better position to buy these things and distribute them to their hospitals.

The attempt to get hospitals NIMS compliant was a slow and painful process. Early practices of compliance "self-reporting" without follow-up verifications at state and federal levels have been troublesome. Some healthcare State level trade organizations openly petitioned against acceptance of preparedness funds, which had state matching fund obligations.

The American College of Healthcare Executives (ACHE), the most powerful and influential healthcare executive educational organization in the nation, failed to advocate for all-hazards readiness and opted to let other trade organizations pick up the gauntlet. Failure in early attempts to attract its membership into all-hazards professional education programs discouraged any meaningful future offerings.

For the last four survey years, members (hospital CEOs) have shown little collective interest in all-hazards issues. Asked to identify their top financial and/or operational issues, disaster preparedness failed to make the top ten. Results in "top CEO issues 2009" found their top three issues, in descending order: financial challenges 76%; healthcare reform implications 63%; patient safety and quality 32%. And at the bottom was disaster preparedness 1%. How would you design your educational program?

These are not your run-of-the-mill healthcare executives. They are today's hospital leaders. Patients depend on them to provide for a safe healthcare environment. Employees depend on them to keep them safe from workplace hazards. Investors depend on them for fiscal stewardship. Board members depend on them to protect their reputation and keep them out of jail. Communities depend on them to make the difference between life and death in times of crisis. In many communities where hospitals are dominant employers, their future economic existence depends on informed decisions by hospital authorities.

The ultimate responsibility for safety and security for all hospital stakeholders is with the hospital board. The board delegates the day-to-day operations to the administrator. At the end of the day, the board retains the duty of care responsibility for quality care and safety for all.

A recent review of a 2007 publication designed to alert hospital boards on serious healthcare quality and safety issues is a good example of denial and disinterest in all-hazards readiness. Getting the Board on Board – What Your Board Needs to Know about Quality and Safety devotes less than one page out of 104 pages on emergency management.

Dealing with issues of quality and safety during periods of routine care is important, but providing a measure of quality and safety during a crisis is the real test of stewardship. The book's glossary and index are silent on the existence of a national strategy for homeland security healthcare readiness.

Recent publication in the industry's Trustee magazine, which is targeted at hospital board members, has an 11-page article entitled, "2010 AHA (American Hospital Association) Environmental Scan (Hot Topics)." Subject issues range across ten broad categories:

1.   Information Technology & E-Health
2.   Insurance Coverage
3.   Political Issues
4.   Provider Organizations & Physicians
5.   Quality & Patient Safety
6.   Science & Technology
7.   Human Resources

8. Consumers & Demographics
9. Economy & Finance
10. Associations

It is difficult to believe that this article in a national hospital <u>Trustee</u> board publication did not consider all-hazards events as worthy of a discussion in an article purported to provide insight and information about market forces having a high probability of affecting the healthcare field. Additional expert commentary which followed seemed satisfied that the environment scan seemed comprehensive.

Traveling the last mile to a viable national response of homeland security healthcare readiness requires harmonizing the efforts of organizations with disparate views of personal and professional success. Traditional first responders view risk as somewhat removed from that of a chief financial officer of a local hospital, much in the same way as the nation's healthcare design and construction professionals and green groups view the all-hazards issue through a different prism. The professional healthcare media is not much help with changing the direction for a more robust workplace. The last three major articles on "hospitals of the future" were devoid of any concern for facility/physical protection.

A leading organization in the community of healthcare risk management is in locked step with the rest of the industry. The American Society for Healthcare Risk Management (ASHRM) <u>Risk Management Handbook for Healthcare Organizations</u> has few details on healthcare organizations' expected role in homeland security. It gives short shrift to the national response framework and the importance of homeland security presidential directives.

The all-hazards threat issue rarely sees the light of day in their many educational programs and enjoys little attention in their major conference events. One would think that

ASHRM would be the place to seek guidance on such issues. A very good place to start would be a conference to address, "What are the consequences of failure to prepare and respond to known threats to patient populations?"

We authored an article in ASHRM Journal in 2005, "Critical issues for homeland security in healthcare sector readiness," and at the same time I surfaced concern over the lack of coverage for the national strategy for homeland security in the existing <u>Risk Management Handbook, Fourth Edition</u>. The Fifth Edition published in 2007 shows little improvement in content associated with national response framework or national incident management systems, which is so critical to any future homeland security healthcare protection.

The Department of Homeland Security Risk Lexicon focuses on the management of meaning and concepts of <u>risk</u> and attempts to provide a single definition for each term. Some aspects of "risk" hold implicit meaning that one would knowingly, not unwittingly, risk a patient population to known death and injury. Is there a place in hospital stewardship to indulge in "risk tolerance," or risk acceptance, when the acceptance of that risk is based on competing "return on investment"?

The last of the 2004, 9/11 Commission recommendations were implemented through Public Law 110-53, Recommendations of the 9/11 Commission Act of 2007. The original recommendations from #26 dealt with the adoption of Instant Command System (ICS) and #28, endorsing private sector adoption of the American National Standards Institute's (ANSI) standards for private preparedness, including the statement:

"We also encourage the insurance and credit-rating industries to look closely at a company's compliance with ANSI standard in assessing its insurability and creditworthiness.

We believe that compliance with the standard should define the standard of care owed by a company to its employees and the public for legal purposes. Private-sector preparedness is not a luxury; it is the cost of doing business in a post 9/11 world. It is ignored at tremendous potential cost in lives, money, and national security."

We find little to no evidence the nation's healthcare insurance industry consistently factors this homeland security ideal into their hospital insurance coverage. The same may be said of the nation's credit lending institutions, both federal and non-federal.

Healthcare accreditation organizations abound. Wikipedia provides a quick look at these organizations. We characterized them as "alphabet soup" (HFAP, JC, NCQA, CHAP, ACHP, HQAA, AAAHC, DNV, etc.) of external evaluation mechanisms.

None of the currently existing hospital external evaluation mechanisms for healthcare emergency management have yet developed assessment schemes which approximate an acceptable level of readiness envisioned by the National Response Framework.

The author has been professionally engaged on one side or the other with healthcare external evaluations for more than 40 years. Established standards of care are designed to ensure a safe and secure patient environment, whether one is faced with earthquakes, floods, forest fires as was the case in Fairbanks, Alaska at -50 degrees, or dust storms, or terrorist attacks at +130 degrees in the desserts of Saudi Arabia. Most of us who are more than casual observers to evolving changes to standards over time understand that survey standards are subject to change as the treatment environment changes.

Many scholars have observed the harmful effects of the "industry to government regulator" swinging door. As we have seen, this leads to egregious conflicts of interest and other actions harmful to the trusting public. There are also concerns over the private sector bodies and the reality of their ability to balance the needs of the industry and the best interest of those receiving their services. These concerns were alive and well long before IOM's landmark "To err is human," probably best articulated by long-time critics and observers of the extant mechanisms for healthcare oversight. The following two quotes are taken from the Presidential Advisory Commission on Consumer Protection's final meeting, March 1998.

"Conflicts of interest can arise from multiple sources. For example, private sector accrediting bodies have, as one of their customers, the entities that the organization accredits. The organizations to be accredited sometimes are the same organizations that created or fostered the creation of the accrediting entity, and often are necessarily

involved in identifying the standards to which they will be held accountable."

"Quality oversight organizations also have a second set of customers – healthcare consumers – who depend on the work of these organizations to make comparative judgments about the quality of certain types of healthcare organizations. This is particularly true when public regulators use accreditation as a means of meeting public standards (e.g., when JCAHO accredited hospitals are deemed to have met Medicare Conditions of Participation). Consumer advocacy organizations become concerned when the accrediting organization seems overly solicitous of the views of the industry, or when very few organizations have their accreditation denied."

The above referenced JCAHO is the re-branded JC, or Joint Commission. This organization has enjoyed a near monopoly in the hospital external evaluation arena and is used extensively as the mechanism of choice to assess healthcare quality, safety and security in the nation's worldwide military, veterans, Native American, and public/private facilities.

The effectiveness of the accreditation and deeming mechanisms on the quality of care measured by hospital acquired infections, treatment errors, and violence in the workplace speak for themselves.

Our attention is focused on "the other side of safety and security, all-hazards readiness." It should be obvious to all that the process did little to protect patients from the ravages of Katrina. The response to 9/11 exposed the gaps in the industry's ability to protect the integrity of the hospital internal space. A quick look back at recent history of what appears to be a movement toward a "culture of preparedness" is in question.

A year before the 9/11 attacks, key

elements of the private/public and governmental healthcare sectors met to consider how best to prepare for and respond to looming threats which would call for a "mass casualty" response from the industry. The broad consensus was to follow the JCAHO 1998 Environment of Care Standards and expand involvement with the greater community. This was followed by a number of public policy initiatives promoting community-wide emergency management.

Fast-forward to June 2007. The Joint Commission alerted the industry that effective January 2008, hospitals were to meet "six critical areas of emergency management." These new "Elements of Performance (EP)" were fundamental to any meaningful decision-making on "to protect in place or evacuate." The pushback from client hospitals and trade organizations intensified, and by the end of the first quarter of the calendar year 2008, these EPs were no longer scored for that year.

We see evidence that critical all-hazards evaluation tools have been formally de-emphasized in 2010 Emergency Management and Environment of Care guidelines. One such process tool useful in reviewing emergency preparedness is the "formal emergency management tracer." This procedure follows the "clinical care tracer" model, which is highly regarded in evaluating quality of care given at various levels and locations of care provided throughout the patient's stay in the hospital. Loss of the formal tracer tool is unfortunate, additionally the removal of key documented "measures of success" requirement further erodes meaningful oversight.

Then there are the "alerts" to the industry which have us scratching our heads. One such "heads-up" alert is the article, "Annual security assessments become California law," which in part states: "California, often the forerunner in compliance standards, may be leading the pack when it comes to security assessments." The law may be unique, but the requirement has been on the books for decades.

The growth of external threats and poor preparedness and response performances in recent all-hazards events on the Gulf Coast and the lack of preparedness for H1N1 pandemic are, at least in part, reflective of a systemic failure of extant external evaluation mechanisms. The vulnerability of hospitals to both inside and outside attacks has increased over the last decade. We see a workplace struggling to deal with hospital acquired infections and seemingly unprepared to protect its own workforce from its own workforce, and one that has minimized the need to defend their organizations from known man-made threats.

"In the Line of Fire – Could Mumbai Happen Again?"

"Mexican Drug Cartels and Hezbollah Operating in Mexico and U.S."

"Chicago Suspect Linked to Mumbai Attacks"

"Santa Cruz Fire Bombs Look Familiar"

"Lawyer: L-1 Visas Used to Dodge H1B Regulations"

"Many California Health Workers Not Checked for Criminal Past"

"Now Labeled a Pandemic, Swine Flu Poses a Threat to Healthcare Workers"

"Hate Group Numbers Up by 50% Since 2000"

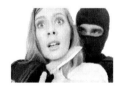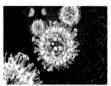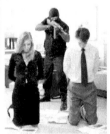

CHAPTER 8: MYTH 8

Hospital Stakeholders are Safe and Secure
in their Hospitals.

Reality: Hospitals are very dangerous places for all employees, in general, and women in particular. The risk of being in an unhealthy environment does not stop with exposure to a whole range of diseases. Female healthcare employees are counted among the most physically assaulted workers in the American workforce.

Violence in hospitals is viewed as a multidimensional problem. The level of violence in the nation's emergency department has risen unabated over the last decade. Hospitals' emergency departments are the hospital's "window to the world" and the door through which some of the most anxious and fearful populations enter.

The triage process makes a lot of sense to those engaged in the activity, but often it is not commonly understood nor shared by patient populations. Increased overcrowding and long waits for treatment elicit strong emotional responses from patients and their families. Even with adequately staffed, skilled security personnel and sufficient numbers of experienced caregivers, treatment sites get overwhelmed.

The lack of available beds for timely admissions for seriously ill patients leads to frustration, and families may lash out at caregivers or become behavioral problems themselves. Many walk-in patients have chronic mental health problems and are often disruptive, loud and aggressive. Gang-related shootings may bring in both the shooters and the victims.

Add the ever-present "forensic patient," who may be a danger to himself or others, with police escort and who also may be a flight risk. Escort officers may or may not be experienced and are often inattentive.

Under the category of "no good deed goes unpunished," anecdotal reports are starting to surface from healthcare organizations that uninsured patients are showing up at physicians' offices and emergency rooms demanding care, now that the healthcare reform bill has been signed into law.

Weapons of every type and description find their way into these treatment sites. Design and construction of facilities do much to mitigate problems associated with space and segregation of unruly patients. Metal detectors are in use by many hospitals across the nation. Hospital authorities are reluctant to employ these proven tools in the fight against violence out of concern for symbolic appearances of an unsafe environment for customers. Security officials find it a hard sell.

One hospital security official tells of a situation where he convinced his executive suite to try a temporary metal detector only at the emergency room entrance. The first month's yield of weapons was more than 500. They included firearms, knives, razors, pepper spray, and an assorted number of items which were designed to inflict harm. Needless to say, metal detectors were to be a permanent fixture in a number of places on this campus.

When interviewing caregivers about "violence in hospitals," the emergency department is generally first to be mentioned. Incident reports tell a broader story. Verbal abuse is recorded from all locations in the hospital; however, physical abuse is always underreported. One-on-one encounters without witnesses are difficult to judge. Violence between and among coworkers is on the rise.

One narrow point in the funnel is Human Resources and a comprehensive criminal background check policy. A recent statewide study of background checks for healthcare workers revealed that one-third of the state's caregivers did not have a criminal background check at the time of employment. The unsettling aspect of this population is that they were caregivers with close person-to-person patient contact relationships; 75% of all psychiatric technicians, 50% of all family therapists, social workers and dentists, and 12% of all physicians.

We now turn to patients as victims of violence from caregivers. One startling report covering the period 1970 to 2006 identified 54 caregivers responsible for over 2,100 deaths. Caregivers who are serial killers have been able to move from hospital to hospital with relative ease. Obviously, the importance of identifying and reporting these offenders should be an organizational priority. One well-intended step taken by the healthcare industry has been to inform the federal government when they take action against dangerous caregivers. The value of having a central registry to protect vulnerable patients across the nation speaks for itself.

The Department of Health and Human Services revealed that its two decade-old national database listing the names of those who were reported as offenders (nurses, pharmacists, psychologists, other healthcare professionals) across the nation "is missing." It provides little comfort to know that they will reconstitute the list as soon as possible. To err is human, but what are the consequences?

Now we will take a look at a new source of human threats to hospitals with which they have limited experience, "The changing face of terrorism and terrorist actors."

Along with the anti-counterterrorism community, many of us were surprised by the active participation of physicians as suicide bombers. Physicians have long held high-ranking leadership roles in various terrorist organizations and have been instrumental in recruiting and sending "foot soldiers out to blow themselves up." Osama bin Laden's second in command, Dr. al-Zawahiri, is a pediatrician.

Events involving physicians as suicide bombers pose a new set of concerns for the international healthcare industry and others. The recent attack on a group of CIA operatives in Afghanistan was carried out by a Jordanian physician. There is little need to discuss the Fort Hood attack.

Shortly after the United Kingdom physician bomber event, the international healthcare and national security organizations engaged in a "deep look-back" and background checks on international medical graduates working abroad. Little open source information has been released about this for potential terrorists within this population. However, the investigators were stunned by the magnitude of false information which surfaced in the form of forged degrees, undocumented professional experience, and nonexistent references.

According to a recent report from the Department of Homeland Security, there are wholesale abuses in the U.S. visa system. The lack of integrity in our visa system is a danger to all work sites. Setting aside the terrorist threat, the danger to patient populations exposed to practitioners who have misrepresented their professional training and experience should be a concern to all.

International medical graduates (IMGs) constituted 27% of the U.S. physician workforce in 2006. Experts tell us that domestic production of physicians and other healthcare professionals will not meet the future needs of known growing demands for healthcare. This will lead to increased recruiting of IMGs. The industry is faced with the need to effectively plan for the potential increase in insider threats posed by this reality.

Experts suggest there may be a shift away from internationally launched terrorist attacks to establish terrorist groups in the United States. The entry of women seeking equal rights as suicide bombers substantially increases the threat population. Domestic terrorists, anti-groups, animal protection, and anti-abortion pose a particular concern for healthcare organizations.

Increased nuclear and biological research on university campuses and medical centers across the nation has ignited a revival of many "anti" groups. The recent surge in hate groups adds to this mix. In effect, they have the same access to materials to "dirty bombs," high-yield explosives, and radioactive material as others who would do us harm.

The old excuses that "our hospital will never be subject to a WMD attack" and "we see no real need to prepare for such an event" ring hollow in the face of the changing terrorist threat landscape. Mumbai's deadly hospital attack was executed by a small number of young men with limited training and armed with conventional weapons. It does not seem unreasonable that such groups could be put together relatively quickly and attack what they believe is a soft target in the community.

SUMMARY

Existing national efforts to protect patients from unnecessary death arising from healthcare acquired infections and treatment errors should be a priority health policy. Promoting a healthy insurance system which provides equitable access to quality care is a noble and just healthcare policy goal. Reduction of aggregated healthcare costs of such expanded care is critical to a sustainable healthcare system.

Lost in the passionate advocacy for these important policy pursuits in the healthcare system is the reality that the value of these achievements would pale by comparison in a multiple flash-bang of nuclear or dirty bomb explosion, or slippage of the Pacific seismic plate, or a raging virulent pandemic.

There are scattered "islands of excellence," where hospital authorities and their communities have taken care to protect their stakeholders. However, the vast majority of hospitals across the nation have failed to "step up to the plate" and address their roles and responsibilities for healthcare security readiness. Under the category of "better late than never" is the <u>National Health Security Strategy of the United States of America</u>, touted as the nation's first National Health Security Strategy (NHSS).

There was a time in the mid-twentieth century when hospitals and healthcare systems fully partnered with civil and military authorities in WMD preparedness and response efforts. To "protect in place" was not for days, but months. To "evacuate" was not only being prepared to "lift stranded groups of seriously ill patients from disabled hospitals," but also to prepare to move entire populations out of harm's way.

A quick review of the guidance to the healthcare industry over the last two decades is a stretch of the imagination to characterize the National Health Security Strategy (NHSS) as the "first call to healthcare industry to prepare for all-hazards readiness." Instead, it is more like the most recent attempt to reorganize past failed attempts to rally the non-federal hospital and healthcare sector to "voluntarily" meet its basic obligations to prepare for homeland security protection.

Failure to protect a trusting public from all-hazards has no political parent. Both political parties are equal opportunity neglectors.

Over the years, we have seen reams of partisan reports identifying what the previous administration has failed to do to protect the public from known threats. (So much for not knowing what had not been done.) Then, when faced with the reality of how difficult it is to move established power brokers, they attach the blinders.

Terrorist groups have little need to employ 17th Street lobbyists or to be creative in their quest to do us harm. They have a cafeteria style menu from which to choose.

Consider the specter of an ambulance loaded to the ceiling with 1,000 pounds of explosives, mixed with generous amounts of radioactive materials pulling up to an emergency entrance, and the driver ignites the bomb.

Consider a VIP limo, its windows darkened, also loaded with 1,500 pounds of explosives, heavily laden and integrated with ten-penny nails and ball bearings pulling up to the entrance of the hospital, which has attracted large numbers of employees expecting a visit from some celebrity, exploding as the door triggers the bomb.

Consider a woman pushing a wheelchair patient into the great glass atrium and igniting a concealed bomb.

Consider a uniformed utility repairman arriving with his equipment bag to repair a malfunctioning air-conditioning system. In his utility bag he has two cylinders of weaponized anthrax, which he skillfully introduces into the HVAC system.

Consider a parcel delivery person has an emergency delivery to the nuclear medicine clinic. It is a large cargo box with "Urgent" written on the top of the box. It appears heavy for one man to carry, so the guard brings a hand truck for its movement, the hand truck pushed into the cesium 137 blood irradiator storage unit. Attached to the package is a timer, which is timed to explode a potential dirty bomb in 30 minutes.

Consider late at night a lonely mortuary vehicle backs up to the morgue door and gets staff to help the driver unload two very heavy caskets. No one notices that they should be empty coming into the hospital. These are only a few from Menu A.

Designing realistic response scenarios on which to exercise mass casualty triage is relatively easy. Crisp detail protocols staffed with your best and brightest are only effective in a protective physical environment in which staff are safe and supplies secure. Crowd control is often overlooked in planning all-hazards events. Had there been a chemical, biological, radiological attack in tandem with the 9/11 terrorist attacks, the lack of crowd control and porous hospital security would have resulted in contamination of existing healthcare resources.

We have been faced with multiple natural disasters in recent years and, with notable exceptions, responded reasonably well.

Managing CBNRE risk requires the understanding of differences between natural and man-made events. With the exception of earthquakes (even then, we know what is happening when it happens), most natural disasters are known in advance; in some cases brief notices, but enough to take steps to defend ourselves. Man-made events are difficult in predictability, casualty production, ratio between property loss and loss of lives, loss of periods of personal freedom, and recovery time.

Bioterrorism is considered among the most pernicious of these threats. They are often in the environment well before they are detected, and the interval between exposure and detection could well spell the difference between life and death.

Experience has shown us that there are substantial differences between and among local hospital preparedness across the country. No one has the corner on the blame. Congressional and federal oversight is spotty. Many states have neglected to pass needed enabling laws which remove serious barriers to an effective response system. Apathy, denial, as well as "cognitive dissonance" from other quarters ring hollow in standing up to the world of "<u>to err is human</u>."

Along the continuum of human errors are legitimate mistakes and a range of "sins of commission" and "sins of omission." From where I sit, "sins of omission" are often the most harmful to the public good, and take less courage.

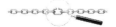

Public Health and Healthcare Sector: The Weakest Link in the Homeland Security Chain?

RECENT PUBLICATIONS

"Homeland Security CBRNE and All-Hazards Healthcare Readiness"

1. Blair, J.D., **All-Hazards "HVA" for Non-Federal Healthcare CBRNE Readiness: A Level Playing Field?** Inside Homeland Security, Volume 3, Issue 5, Sept/Oct 2005.

2. Blair, J.D., **Homeland Security and the Non-Federal Healthcare Sector: Evaluation of Your Incident Command System (ICS),** Journal of Healthcare Protection Management, Volume 21, Number 2, Summer 2005.

3. Blair, J.D**., Homeland Security and Non-Federal Health Sector: Incident Command Structure.** Hospital Fire Marshal's News (HFMA), April 2005.

4. Blair, J.D., **National Response Plan and the Non-Federal Healthcare Industry's Design and Construction Community**, Matrix, 2005.
5. Blair, J.D., **Healthcare Readiness for CBRNE Terrorist Events, Emergency Response Manual, Chapter 25,** Anti-Terrorism Board Certified Anti-Terrorism

Specialist (ATAB).

6. Blair, J.D., Edwards, J. T., **Critical Issues for Homeland Security and Healthcare Readiness**, Journal of Healthcare Risk Management, October 2005.

7. Blair, J.D., **Is Healthcare the Weak Link in the Homeland Security Chain?** Medical News, January 2006, KY Medical News (KY, IN, OH).

8. Blair, J.D., **Homeland Security and the Non-Federal Sector Readiness**. Hospital Fire Marshal's Association, Part 1, December 2005, Part 2, January 2006.

9. Blair, J.D., **Perspectives on Advanced Directives, Monograph,** Task Force Member, American Society for Healthcare Risk Management, August 2006.

10. Blair, J.D., **Is The Healthcare Industry Prepared for Terrorism?** Journal of Healthcare Protection Management, Volume 22, Number 1.

11. Blair, J.D., Silver, R. B., Modern Healthcare, **"Commentary"** Daily Dose and Modern Healthcare Online, January 2007.

12. Blair, J.D., Scanlon, P. A., **Pandemic Flu Threat and Business Continuity.** Elliot Consulting Group, News Letter.

13. Blair, J.D., Dluzneski, P. K., **Evolving Roles and Responsibilities for Healthcare Security Professionals: The Non-Federal Healthcare Sector Meets NIMS and NIPP,** Journal of Healthcare Protection Management, January 2007.

14. Blair, J.D., **NIPPS vs. Non-Federal Hospital Design and Construction**, Letter to the Editor, Health Affairs, July 2006.

15. Blair, J.D., **Lagging Healthcare Sector,"** Updates and Responses, *HSToday.us*, April 2007.

16. Blair, J.D., **"Are Medical Facilities Doing Enough to Prepare for Catastrophic Events?"** Healthcare Construction and Operation, March 2008.

17. Blair, J.D., Scanlon, P. A., **Reflections on a "Motto,"** Hospital Fire Marshals Association, HFMA NEWS, September 2008.

18. Blair, J.D., Scanlon, P. A., Dluzneski, P.D., **To Protect in Place or Evacuate? That is the Question,** Journal of Health Protection Management, Volume 24, Number 2, September 2008.

19. Blair, J.D., **Is the Healthcare Industry Prepared for Terrorism? Revisited,** Inside Homeland Security, Volume 7, Issue 1, Spring 2009.

20. Blair, J.D., **GITMO Detainees and U.S. Host Communities: Is Your Hospital Prepared to Live with Terrorist Inmates in Your Backyard?** Journal of Healthcare Protection Management, Volume 25, Number 2, Summer 2009.

21. Blair, J.D., **GITMO Detainees and U.S. Host Communities: Is Your Hospital Prepared to Live with Terrorist Inmates in Your Backyard?** Inside Homeland

Security, Volume 7, Issue 4, Winter 2009.

22. Blair, J.D., **James D. Blair On What Hospitals Can Do To Overcome Deficiencies in All-Hazards Preparedness, IAHSS Directions,** Volume 21, Number 3, 2008 Journal.

REFERENCES

Guide to Emergency Management and Related Terms, Definitions, Concepts, Acronyms, Organisms, Programs, Guidance and Legislation,
B. Wayne Blanchard, Ph.D., CEM
January 22, 2008
(Date of Last Modification)

The U.S. Government Accountability Office (GAO) is an independent, nonpartisan agency that works for Congress. Often called the "congressional watchdog," GAO investigates how the federal government spends taxpayer dollars. The GAO responds to requests from Congress and their products back to the Congress to answer specific questions asked by the body. As you will see in the GAO Reports, they have dutifully reported on requested areas of investigation. The scope of the GAO's investigations is limited to carefully worded requests. GAO contacts explain that resources also serve as a barrier to more comprehensive coverage of issues. Specific reports include:

GAO-06-826 – Disaster Preparedness: Limitations in Federal Evacuation Assistance for Health Facilities Should be Addressed

GAO-07-1253t – September 11: Problems Remain in Planning for and Providing Health Screening and Monitoring Services for Responders

GAO-08-610 – September 11: HHS Needs to Develop a Plan that Incorporates Lessons from the Responder Health Programs

GAO-04-850 – Medicare: CMS Needs Additional Authority to Adequately Oversee Patient Safety in Hospitals

GAO-10-381t – Emergency Preparedness: State Efforts to Plan for Medical Surge Could Benefit from Shared Guidance for Allocating Scarce Medical Resources

GAO-02-150t – Homeland Security: Key Elements of a Risk Management Approach
GAO-03-233 – Critical Infrastructure

Protection: Challenges for Selected Agencies and Industry Sectors

GAO-07-833t – Homeland Security: Management and Programmatic Challenges Facing the Department of Homeland Security

GAO-07-39 – Critical Infrastructure Protection: Progress Coordinating Government and Private Sector Efforts Varies by Sectors' Characteristics

GAO-07-706r – Critical Infrastructure Protection: Sector Plans and Sector Council Continue to Evolve

GAO-10-60 – Centers for Medicare and Medicaid Services: Deficiencies in Contract Management Internal Control are Pervasive

GAO-08-539 – Influenza Pandemic: Federal Agencies Should Continue to Assist States to Address Gaps in Pandemic Planning

GAO-07-395t – Homeland Security: Preparing

for and Responding to Disasters

GAO-09-828 – **Homeland Defense**: Greater Focus on Analysis of Alternatives and Threats Needed to Improve DOD's Strategic Nuclear Weapons Security

GAO-09-909t – **Influenza Pandemic**: Gaps in Pandemic Planning and Preparedness Need to be Addressed

GAO-06-433r – **Coast Guard**: Deployable Operations Group Achieving Organizational Benefits, but Challenges Remain

GAO-02-141t – **Bioterrorism**: Public Health and Medical Preparedness

GAO-08-39 – **Stabilization and Reconstruction**: Actions are Needed to Develop a Planning and Coordination Framework and Establish Civilian Reserve Corps

GAO-08-36 – **Influenza Pandemic**:

Opportunities Exist to Address Critical Infrastructure Protection Challenges that Require Federal and Private Sector Coordination

GAO-08-369 – National Disaster Response: FEMA Should Take Action to Improve Capacity and Coordination between Government and Voluntary Sectors

GAO-08-668 – Emergency Preparedness: States are Planning for Medical Surge, but Could Benefit from Shared Guidance for Allocating Scarce Medical Resources

GAO-08-768 – National Response Framework: FEMA Needs Policies and Procedures to Better Integrate Non-Federal Stakeholders in the Revision Process

GAO-08-808 – Health-Care-Associated Infections in Hospitals: An Overview of State Reporting Programs and Individual Hospital Initiatives to Reduce Certain Infections

GAO-08-334 – **Influenza Pandemic**: Sustaining Focus on the Nation's Planning and Preparedness Efforts

GAO-08-960t – **Biosurveillance**: Preliminary Observations on Department of Homeland Security's Biosurveillance Initiatives

GAO-08-919r – **Initial Results** on Availability of Terrorism Insurance in Specific Geographic Markets

GAO-07-706r – **Critical Infrastructure Protection**: Sector Plans and Sector Councils Continue to Evolve

GAO-10-73 – **Influenza Pandemic**: Monitoring and Assessing the Status of the National Pandemic Implementation Plan Needs Improvement

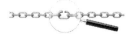

The Congressional Research Service (CRS) serves shared staff to congressional committees and Members of Congress. CRS experts assist at every stage of the legislative process – from the early considerations that precede bill drafting, through committee hearings and floor debate, to the oversight of enacted laws and various agency activities. Reference documents include:

CRS-r40159 – Federal Efforts to Address the Threat of Bioterrorism: Selected Issues for Congress

CRS-rl31225 – Bioterrorism: Summary of a CRS/National Health Policy Forum Seminar on Federal, State, and Local Public Health Preparedness

CRS-rl34724 – Would an Influenza Pandemic Qualify as a Major Disaster Under the Stafford Act?

CRS-rl33053 – Federal Stafford Act Disaster Assistance: Presidential Declarations, Eligible Activities, and Funding

NON-AUTHOR BOOKS

Jordan, M., P.h.D., *Nursing in Hell: The Katrina Experience*, Lambert Academic Publishing, November 2009.

Joint Commission Resources, *Getting the Board on Board: What Your Board Needs to Know About Quality and Patient Safety*, 2007.

Ramsey, D. A., Rush, J., *Unprepared*, Daydreamer Books, 2010.

Diaz, T., Newman, B., *Lightning Out of Lebanon: Hezbollah Terrorists on American Soil*, Ballantine Books, 2005.

Natural Disasters: Protecting the Public's Health, Pan American Health Organization, Scientific Publication No-575.

Management of Dead Bodies after Disasters, Field Manual 2006.

Health Care Facilities Handbook, NFPA 99, 2005 Edition.

Nuclear Radiation Does Not Make You Glow, Prepared by Ecology and Environment, Include., and The Palladino Company, Inc, U. S. Environmental Protection Agency Emergency Response Section, Region 9, 2007.

Humanitarian Supply Management and Logistics in the Health Sector, Pan American Health Organization 2001.

OSHA Reference Guide, What You Need to Know in Healthcare, HCPro, Inc., 2004.

American Board for Certification in Homeland Security, Copy National Response Framework, January 2009.

Dorin, A. F., *Jihad and American Medicine*, Praeger Security International, November 2008.

Gabriel, B., *They Must Be Stopped*, St. Martin's Press, N.Y., September 2008.

Gingrich, N., Pavey, D., Woodbury, A., *Saving Lives & Saving Money*, Gingrich Communications, Inc., 2003.

NON-AUTHOR ARTICLES

Lurie, N., Wasserman, J., Nelson, C. D., "Preparedness: Evolution or Revolution?" *Health Affairs*, July/August 2005, Volume 25, Number 4.

Moore, M., "Vigilance Reduces Vulnerabilities - Protect Your Hospital," *MATRIX*, Volume 2, Issue 2.

Shadden, M., "Planning to Survive and Operate: Business Continuity," *Inside Homeland Security*, Volume 7, Issue 1, Spring 2009.

Gabriel, B., "The Enemy Next Door: Terrorists Among Us," *Inside Homeland Security*, Volume 7, Issue 4, Winter 2009.

Michelman, B. S., "The Amazing Evolution of an Industry: Past, Present and Future of Healthcare Security," *Journal of Healthcare Protection Management*, Volume 20, Number 1, Winter 2002.

McLaughlin, S., Spaanbroek, S., "We'll figure out what to do when the time comes: the need for developing effective emergency operation exercises," *Journal of Healthcare Protection Management*, Volume 25, Number 1, 2009.

Williams, J. T., "Suicide bombers: Are you a target? What can you do?" *Journal of Healthcare Protection Management,* Volume 22, Number 2, 2006.

Huser, T. J., "Suspect SARS patient puts hospital's plan on defense," *Journal of Healthcare Protection Management*, Volume 21, Number 1, Winter 2005.

Perry, R. W., Lindell, M. K., "Hospital Planning for Weapons of Mass Destruction," *Journal of Healthcare Protection Management*, Volume 23, Number 1, 2007.

Gacki-Smith, J., Juarez, A. M., Boyett, L., Homeyer, C., Robinson, L., MacLean, S. L., "Violence Against Nurses Working in U.S. Emergency Departments," *Journal of Healthcare Protection Management*, Volume 26, 2010;26(1):81-99.

Yoker, B. C., Kizer, K. W., Lampe, P., Forrest, A. R. W., Lannan, J. M., Russell, D. A., "Serial Murder by Healthcare Professionals," *Journal of Healthcare Protection Management*, Volume 24, Number 1, 2008.

Pettit, W. R., "Prepare Now for Pandemic Readiness Security and Patient Surge," *Journal of Healthcare Protection Management*, Volume25, Number 2, 2009.

Spencer, P., "The Security Case for Patient and Family Centered Care," *Journal of Healthcare Protection Management*, Volume 24, Number 2, 2008.

Elzer, R. M., "Guide to CMS Compliance," *Journal of Healthcare Management*, Volume 55, Number 2, March/April 2010.

Robinson, L. A., Hammitt, J. K., Aldy, J. E., Krupnick, A., Baxter, J., "Valuing the Risk of Death from Terrorist Attacks," *Journal of Homeland Security and Emergency Management*, Volume 7, Issue 1, Article 14, 2010.

CDC Center for Disease Control and Prevention H1N1 Flu, "Interim Guidance for Correctional and Detention Facilities on Novel Influenza A (H1N1) Virus," *CDC.gov*, May 24, 2009.

Chambers, H., "Construction: 8 Complexes are Unsafe, According to State," *San Diego Business Journal*, April 19, 2010.

"FBI, nuclear agency investigates terrorism suspect," *CNN.com,* March 12, 2010.

Associated Press: "Study: Terrorists shifting focus to 'soft' targets," *STRATFOR.com* report, September 8, 2009.

Zigmond, J., "Extreme Makeover, HHS should offer more emergency guidance: GAO," *ModernHealthcare.com*, February 1, 2010.

Kauffman, T., "Plutonium spill, laser accident prompt reviews," *FederalTimes.com*, September 7, 2008.

Bender, B., "Security specialists say U.S. is more vulnerable to attack," *Boston.com*, September 11, 2008.

Johnson, K., Frank T., "Mumbai attacks refocus U.S. Cities," *USATODAY.com*, December 5, 2008.

Stewart, S., "Dirty Bombs Revisited: Combating the Hype," *STRATFOR.com*, April 22, 2010.

Kliff, S., Skipp, C., "Overlooked: The Littlest Evacuees," *Newsweek*, October 6, 2008.

Blesch, G., "Hospital Settles in Katrina-Related Case," *Modern Healthcare*, January 27, 2010.

Hall, M., "Now Labeled a Pandemic, Swine Flu Poses Threat to Healthcare Workers," *AFL-CIO NOW Blog*, June 12, 2009.

Adcox, S., "Nuclear Waste Piles Up at Hospitals," Associated Press, September 26, 2008.

Gorman, S., "Bioterrorism's Threat Persists As Top Security Risk," *Wall Street Journal*, August 4, 2008.

McCarter M., "Dirty Bomb Recovery Plan Lacking," *HSToday.us*, March 1, 2010.

Baldor, L., "Small Terror Groups are Homeland Challenge of Future," *Homeland1.com*, April 2010.

Webster, M., "Mexican Drug Cartel and Hezbollah Operating in Mexico and U.S.," *American Chronicle*, October 26, 2008.

McCarter, M., "Officials Outline Terrorist Threats to United States," *HSToday.us*, October 2, 2009.

Ornstein, C., Webber, T., "Many California Health Workers Not Checked For Criminal Pasts," *L.A. Times*, December 2008.

Ephron, D., Hosenball, M., "Recruited for Jihad? About 20 Young Somali-American Men in Minneapolis Have Recently Vanished," *Newsweek*, February 2, 2009.

Trull, F., "Animal Rights Terrorism, Activists Have Used Increasingly Dangerous Tactics on Researchers Whose Goal is to Save Lives," *L.A. Times*, August 2008.

Thomas G., "MI5 Discover Al-Qaeda Buying Ambulances on Ebay" *G2 Magazine*, November 2008.

Kavilanz, P., "U.S. To hospitals: Clean up your act," *CNN Money.com*, April 2010.

Hoffman, D. E., "The Little Nukes That Got Away," *Foreign Policy.com*, April 2010.

Wallask, S., "Five Lessons U.S. Hospitals Can Take from Haiti," *HealthLeaders Media*, January 2010.

NBC News, "FBI: U.K. terror suspects tried to work in U.S.," July 2007.

Ali Zulfigar., King, L., "Pakistan's Taliban Leader threatens attacks in the U.S.," *L.A. Times*, April 2009.

Hospital Safety Center, HCPro, "Annual security assessments become California law," June 2010.

Joint Commission Online, "Accreditation: Measures of Success requirements deleted," *Joint Commission.org*, April 2010.

Joint Commission, "Hospitals of the Future Report," *Joint Commission.org*, November 2008.

Phares, W., "Warning: The Jihadist are Mushrooming Inside America," *Family Security Matters.org*, September 2009.

Kiltz, L., "Developing Critical Thinking Skills in Homeland Security and Emergency Management Courses," *Journal of Homeland Security and Emergency Management*, Volume 6, Issue 1, 2009.

Burton, L., "The Constitutional Roots of All-Hazards Policy, Management, and Law," The Berkeley Electronic Press, *bepress.com*, 2008.

Ramirez, M., "The Unprepared Beware," *EzineArticles.com*, March 2007.

FEMA, "NIMS Alert: FY 2008 and 2009 NIMS Implementation Objectives for Healthcare Organizations," *fema.gov*, June 2008.

FEMA, "NIMS Alert: The National Preparedness Directorate Release of Public Health and Medical Resource Typing Definitions and Job Titles," *fema.gov,* January 2009.

Clark, C., "10 Years after To Err is Human: Are Hospitals Safer?" *HealthLeaders Media*, November 2009.

California Nurses Association, "Many Hospitals Are Not Ready for H1N1: Nurse Survey Shows Deficiencies in Hospital Swine Flu Readiness," *calnurses.org*, August 2009.

McFee, Dr. Robin, "On Terrorism: WMD Preparedness," *IAHSS Directions*, Volume 22, Number 1, *Journal of Healthcare Protection Management,* 2009.

NON-AUTHOR REPORTS

Jewell, K., McGiffert L., "To Err is Human-To Delay is Deadly," Consumers Union, *Safe Patient Project.org*, May 2009.

U.S. Department of Health and Human Services, "National Health Security Strategy of The United States of America," *hhs.org*. December 2009.

McCaffrey, B. R., "Strategic Challenges Facing the Obama Administration," PDF, *afa.org*, August 2009.

Rogers, M. C., "The Liability Risk of Hospitals as a Target of Terrorism," National Emergency Management Summit, Washington, D.C., February 2008 (Presentation).

Defense Science Board, "Challenges to Military Operations in Support of U. S. Interests," Summer 2007 (Study Report).

Graham, B., Talent, J., "World at Risk: The Report of the Commission on the Prevention of Weapons of Mass Destruction Proliferation and Terrorism," December 2009.

American Hospital Association, Final Report, Summary of an Invitational Forum, "Hospital Preparedness for Mass Casualties," August 2000.

Salinsky, E., "Strong as the Weakest Link: Medical Response to a Catastrophic Event," National Health Policy Forum, Background Paper – No. 65 August 8, 2008.

Southern Poverty Law Center, "Hate Group Numbers Up by 54% Since 2000," February 2009.

9/11 Commission Report, "Final report of the National Commission on Terrorist Attacks Upon the United States," 2004.

Mead, C., Molander, R. C., "Considering the Effects of a Catastrophic Terrorist Attack," RAND Corporation, 2006.

U.S. Hearing: Subcommittee on Oversight and Investigations of the Committee on International Relations, "Visa Overstays: Can We Bar the Terrorist Door?" (109th Congress), May 2006.

U.S. House of Representatives Report 109-377, "A Failure of Initiative: Final Report of the Select Bipartisan Committee to Investigate the Preparedness for and Response to Hurricane Katrina," U.S. House of Representatives, 2006.

GAO-10-436 – Defense Infrastructure (DOD Anti-terrorism Construction Standards: DOD Needs to Determine and Use the Most Economical Building Materials and Methods When Acquiring New Permanent Facilities, April 1020.

Third Way, Center for American Progress Action Fund, "Homeland Security Presidential Transition Initiative," November 2008.

Fluman, A., Sanders, M., "Memorandum to Hospital Administrators, State and Local Emergency Managers and Public Health Directors," NIMS Compliance Activities. May 2006 (Memorandum).

President's Advisory Commission on Consumer Protection in the Health Care Industry, Final Meeting, March 1998.

Bradford, D., "Hospital Liability, Lessons Learned from Katrina, QuickNote, Advisen Ltd., October 2005.

Bradford D., Rubkin B., Viscardi P., White Paper Risk Management Series, "The New World of Extreme Risk: Terrorism Disaster Preparedness," Advisen Ltd., October 2001.

McFee, R., "Exclusive: Doctor Evil? Physicians & Scientists – Terrorists & Murderers in an Era of Global Terrorism" (part Three of Four).

Union (AFL-CIO, AFSCME, AFT, CWA, SEUI, UAN, UFCW) Survey Report, "Healthcare Workers In Peril: Preparing To Protect Worker Health And Safety During Pandemic Influenza," April 2009.

AUTHOR PROFILE

James "Jim" Blair, DPA, MHA, FACHE, FABCHS, is President of the Center for HeathCare Emergency Readiness (CHCER). He is a career-retired Army Colonel with 28 years of active service. His Army staff assignments include Chief of Staff of 7th Medical Command and USAREUR Deputy Chief Surgeon for Medical Support Services. He served in the role of Chief Executive Officer in hospitals ranging from Combat Field and Combat Evacuation, Medical Center, Medical System with two Medical Centers and eleven hospitals. He also holds a number of combat awards.

Among his private sector experiences are Vice President, Hospital Corporation of America (HCA), Middle East Limited, independent consultant to the Joint Commission International, independent healthcare consulting to the Middle East and Africa, and independent consultant to Native American Tribes under the

Indian Sovereignty Act.

His Public Sector experiences include Deputy Director of Operations, South Carolina Heath and Human Services Finance Commission, as well as numerous academic appointments to universities. Dr. Blair is a member of Epsilon Phi Delta National Honor Society in Heath Administration and the author of numerous articles spanning a number of expert domains in healthcare.

Why This Is So Important...

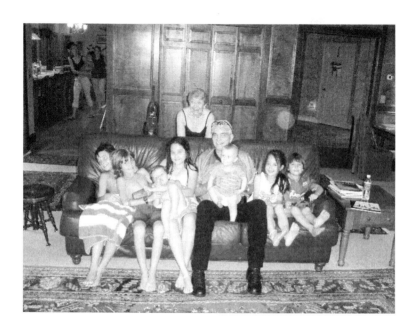